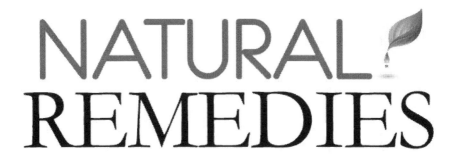

NATURAL REMEDIES

NATURAL REMEDIES THAT HEAL, PROTECT AND PROVIDE INSTANT RELIEF FROM EVERYDAY COMMON AILMENTS

Disclaimer

The information in this book is not to be used as medical advice and is not meant to treat or diagnose medical problems. The information presented should be used in combination with guidance from your physician.

Disclaimer and Terms of Use: Effort has been made to ensure that the information in this book is accurate and complete, however, the author and the publisher do not warrant the accuracy of the information, text and graphics contained within the book due to the rapidly changing nature of science, research, known and unknown facts and internet. The Author and the publisher do not hold any responsibility for errors, omissions or contrary interpretation of the subject matter herein. This book is presented solely for motivational and informational purposes only.

Introduction

The side-effect list at the end of the average medicinal commercial is alarming. In a deep hum-drum voice, the announcer dives into his required inclusion of the intense side effects featured in both prescribed and over-the-counter medications. As the medicine works to annihilate one body ailment, it immediately creates an alarming array of other ailments, bringing a continuous cycle of one medicine after another. And how can you, the consumer, understand precisely how the medicines are made or what each bizarre ingredient refers to? Don't turn a blind, ignorant eye.

Stop the medicinal cycle in its tracks and look to the natural remedies found in your very own kitchen! The natural remedies are cost-effective; they hold none of the advertising, processed nature, or marketing of their counter-productive commercial products. Because one can generally find natural ingredients around the house, natural remedies cost almost nothing. Furthermore, one can understand precisely what goes into the natural remedies. As a general rule, you shouldn't put anything in the body or on the skin that isn't completely understood.

Natural remedies in this book look to soothe common headaches, coughs, colds, toenail fungi, and so many other ailments. Because the ingredients listed in this book are plant-based and natural, they do nothing to irritate or create future problems. In fact, they are generally good for the rest of the body as they enact on the very particular, affected area. Heal your body with fresh, healthy ingredients that work for better over-all health. Something as simple as a flower in the field, a garlic clove, or a bit of honey can stretch a long way in the terms of future wellness.

Make the ultimate switch to prevent future problems, eliminate the surge of chemicals in the body, and supercharge the body with health. Live a fulfilled, longer life. Alleviate headaches, arthritis pain and tension with natural techniques, and calm the mind with homemade remedies so you can rest assured that you are doing all you can to take care of your body and overall health.

Table of Contents

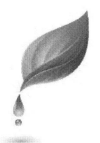

Chapter 1

COMMON, EVERYDAY AILMENT REMEDIES

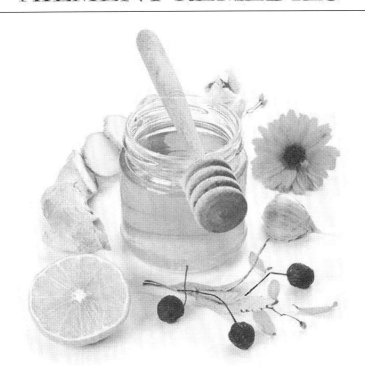

HEAT HEADACHE

Headaches occur when blood vessels in the head expand and push up against nerve endings, resulting in undue pain and unbearable, pounding temples. Headaches traditionally stem from lack of sleep, alcohol consumption, and, quite often, heat and humidity. Heat exhaustion contributes to headaches as well, bringing a pounding head, clammy skin, vomiting, and complete fatigue. Look to the following natural remedies for rejuvenation.

1. Lemon

Drinking a hot cup of lemon tea or simply some hot water with lemon can assist with the reduction of headache pain. The citrus of the lemon reduces the stress associated with the heat headache, and the water can continue to hydrate, thus cooling the intensity of the blood vessels against the nerves.

2. Betel Leaves

Betel leaves have analgesic and cooling properties that assist in the removal of headaches.

Directions:
Place three betel leaves in a food processor or grinder and make a fine paste. Smear the paste on the forehead and on the sides of the head, by the

temples, and allow it to sit for thirty minutes. Meanwhile, chew a few betel leaves to relieve the headache rapidly.

3.Ginger

Ginger has immense anti-inflammatory properties. Furthermore, it relaxes the blood vessels pushing against the nerve endings, and helps reduce the swelling in the brain. It activates natural opiates in the brain as well; this lessens the interior tension.

Directions:
Drink three to four cups of ginger tea during a headache, and begin drinking the tea at the first sign of head tension. The ginger can act quickly and potentially eliminate the highest levels of headache pain.

JOINT PAIN

Movement seems like a given, right? Something so effortless. If someone wants to walk somewhere, pick something up, it's easy. However, joint pain eliminates that freedom. Joint pain stems from inflammation of one or more joints and often comes in the form of arthritis. Two different forms of arthritis, osteo and rheumatoid, affect the joint in unique ways. Osteoarthritis occurs when the cartilage, or the bone protectant, between the bones actually wears down, forcing the bones to grate together. Rheumatoid, however, is caused by an interior auto-immune disorder. Look to the following joint pain remedies for both arthritis and run-of-the-mill joint pain.

1. Epsom Salt Soak

Epsom salt is fueled with magnesium sulfate, a naturally occurring mineral that is utilized to rid the body of pain.

Directions:
Add a half a cup of Epsom salt to a bowl full of warm water. Stir the Epsom salt and then place the painful joints in the water. Allow the joints to soak for fifteen minutes. If, on the other hand, the joint is somewhere inconvenient, like in the knee, consider taking an Epsom salt bath.

2. Turmeric and Ginger Tea

Both ginger and turmeric are anti-inflammatory, natural products that assist with both formations of arthritis. Turmeric's active ingredient is curcumin, an incredible antioxidant that relieves inflamed cells at the joint center.

Directions:
Create a tea by boiling two cups of water in a saucepan. Afterwards, add one half of a teaspoon of both ground ginger and ground turmeric. Allow the water to simmer for fifteen minutes before straining. Drink it slowly with honey, and enjoy it twice every day for maximum benefits.

3. Dandelion Leaves

Dandelions are the occasional nuisances for someone trying to maintain a pretty lawn. However, those yellow "weeds" pack a real punch in their leaves. Their leaves contain vitamin A and vitamin C, and they can repair damaged tissue around the joints. Furthermore, their minerals help alleviate the liver and clear toxins from the blood.

Directions:
Boil one cup of water. Place three teaspoons of fresh dandelion leaves and allow them to sit for five minutes. Afterwards, strain the tea. Drink this mixture twice a day, but add a little honey.

Dandelion leaves are quite bitter.

4. Eucalyptus and Peppermint Oil

Neither peppermint or eucalyptus help to reduce arthritis. However, they do have a hand in eliminating the pain. They produce a cooling sensation that can bring temporary relief.

Directions:

Bring together seven drops of eucalyptus oil and seven drops of peppermint oil. Blend them well. Afterwards, add two tablespoons of carrier oil. This carrier oil dilutes the other oils so as not to irritate the skin cells. Rub the mixture over the joints when they especially ache, and store the mixture in a cool, dark place.

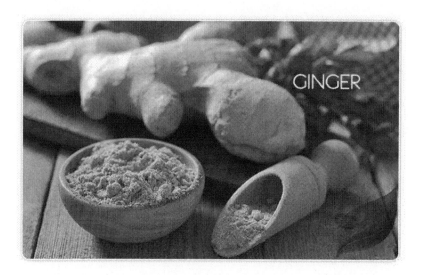

YEAST INFECTION

Yeast infections affect women all over the world with vaginitis: a burning, itching, and painful reaction in the vaginal area. Yeast infections are caused by a wide variety of organisms, and many of these organisms are natural in the environment of the healthy vagina. Generally, the yeast infection culprit is a fungus called Candida albicans. If a doctor has diagnosed a yeast infection, you can look to the following at-home remedies in order to rid yourself of the often embarrassing and irritating yeast infection reactions. However, if the reaction you experience is foul-smelling, frothy, or yellowish, you may be affected with a protozoa called Trichomonas. In that case, you must not move forward with the following home remedies and receive a prescription from a doctor.

1. Yogurt

Yogurt is filled with live cultures that are excellent remedies for yeast infections; they assist the vagina in its restoration of the acid-bacteria balance.

Directions:
You can, of course, eat the yogurt to extinguish the yeast infection problems from the interior. However, utilizing plain yogurt externally works wonders. Place one or two tablespoons into the vagina and also around the exterior, where it's harsh and red.

Alternately, you can utilize the yogurt as a sort of douche by diluting the yogurt with warm water.

2. Drink Cranberry Juice and Munch on Garlic

Cranberry juice without the added sugar acidifies one's vaginal secretion and allows the vaginal secretions to actively fight off the yeast. Furthermore, two fresh garlic cloves a day clear yeast infections with antifungal properties and including garlic in everyday meals prevents the growth of yeast.

3. Apple Cider Vinegar

Apple cider vinegar is one of the strongest natural antibiotics in the world. It kills nearly every bacteria, protozoa, and virus, and it can eliminate candida albicans indefinitely. Furthermore, it can alter the intestines and vagina, charging them with good bacteria that will disallow candida albicans from growing again.

Directions:
There are generally two ways to rid one's self of yeast infection with apple cider vinegar. First, you can drink it every single day. Mix two tablespoons of apple cider vinegar with a glass of water and drink it three times a day. Make sure not to add any sort of sweetener, even honey, as yeast absolutely adores sugar. This is a "rest of life" type of remedy: you are

sure to prevent any future yeast attacks.

Alternately, one can soak a clean cloth in apple cider vinegar and place it around on the vagina, and inside the vagina. Make sure, in this case, that the apple cider vinegar is five percent acidity or less so as to prevent burning.

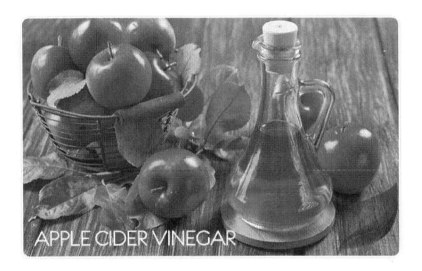

MENSTRUAL CRAMPS

Women plagued with painful periods find themselves aching and popping endless aspirin, waiting for the pain to end. The cramps stem from the uterus shedding its natural lining, forcing the uterine muscle to contract. These contractions force blood vessels to constrict, reducing blood flow and resulting in endless pain. Some women have greater amounts of hormones than others, and therefore they have greater pain. However, natural remedies can help decrease this pain.

1. Raspberry Leaf Tea

Raspberry leaf tea is a mild uterine tonic that helps to reduce pain in the uterine lining. Drink a cup of the raspberry leaf tea every single day of the month to reduce menstrual pain. The tea can be found at a local health food store; however, make sure to look for herbal tea, not black raspberry flavored tea.

2. Reduce Coffee Consumption

Caffeine from coffee is a vasoconstrictor; that is, it forces blood vessels to constrict. Therefore, the blood vessels in the uterine lining may constrict much more in coffee-drinkers than non-coffee drinkers. If coffee is something one cannot give up entirely, it's best to eliminate coffee the week before a period to see a change.

3. Eat Dark, Leafy Greens

Dark, leafy greens are fueled with calcium, magnesium, and other nutrients. The nutrients in these vegetables control muscle contractions. Furthermore, dandelion leaves work as a diuretic and can, therefore, reduce bloating in the lower stomach.

TENDON AND LIGAMENT PAIN

Tendons attach the bone to the muscle, and ligaments attach the bone to the bone. Needless to say, they're pretty important. Pain in the tendons has multiple causes, including: joint strain, tendinitis, and certain illnesses. Much like joint pain, tendon and ligament pain render one useless in general, everyday performances.

1. Arnica Gel

The extracts from yellow blossoms are utilized to make arnica, a homeopathic medication. When rubbed topically, arnica gel works to remedy inflamed tendons. Look to the following recipe to learn DIY arnica gel techniques.

Ingredients:
1 ounce dried arnica herbs
1.5 ounces Beeswax
¾ cup oil with infused arnica
5 drops Wintergreen Essential Oil

Directions:
Begin six weeks before you plan on having the arnica cream on hand. Pour ¾ cup of olive oil, or whatever oil is on hand, in a jar overtop 1 ounce of dried arnica herbs. Shake the jar with the oil and the herbs every single day for six weeks.

After six weeks, place the jar—with the top off—in a

pot of pre-boiling water. Add the beeswax into the oil of the jar and stir well until the beeswax is completely melted. Afterwards, drip five drops of Wintergreen Essential Oil into the jar. Stir well. Remove the jar from the boiling water and allow it to cool. Make sure the container is sealed tight, and store the gel in a cool, dark location. When using, apply the gel over the aching ligament or tendon spots.

2. Calendula Cream

Calendula is actually a marigold flower native to Asia and Europe. Calendula gel or cream, when rubbed topically over the tendon or ligament, is excellent for relieving pain and restoring the body. Most notably, it assists the body with ruptured muscles and tendons. Look to the following DIY recipe to create an at-home tendon and ligament relief cream.

Ingredients for Calendula-Infused Olive Oil:
3 ounces dried calendula herb
1 cup olive oil

Ingredients for Calendula Cream:
2 ounces coconut oil
5 ounces olive oil (infused with the above calendula herb)
2 ounces distilled water
5 drops lavender essential oil

1 tsp. beeswax

Directions:
Place the dried calendula herbs in a small bowl and place that bowl in a pre-boiling pot of water. Pour the olive oil into the bowl and stir briefly. Allow the herbs and oil to heat slowly, keeping the water at around one hundred degrees Fahrenheit. Stir every few minutes for two hours. Afterwards, strain the oil into a jar or container.

Place a different, larger bowl in the pre-boiling pot of water. Add the coconut oil, the beeswax, and the pre-made olive oil. Stir on low heat and allow everything to melt and assimilate together. Remove the bowl from the heated water.

To the side, place water into a blender and whir it for a moment. While the water chugs around the blender, pour the prepared oily and fatty mixture into the blender. Allow the blender to completely mix the ingredients together.

Allow the cream to cool and then apply it to any ligament or tendon areas. Afterwards, store the cream in a cool, dark place. It should keep for up to a year.

3. RhusToxicodendron

RhusToxicodendron is a homeopathic remedy,

otherwise known by its common name, poison ivy. In actuality, rhustoxicodendron is perfect to treat strains, sprains, tendon pain, and ligament pain. It comes in ointment or gel formation, and can be rubbed over the ligament or tendon area to reduce swelling and pain.

Unfortunately, because Rhustox is derived from poison ivy, making a cream at home with a Rhustox base is dangerous and can cause rash. Therefore, look to find Rhustox cream at a local health food store or homeopathy store.

4. Exercise

Exercise seems counterproductive with regards to pain, no? But exercise allows blood flow to the affected joint, bringing nutrients and added oxygen for productive healing. Furthermore, exercise builds strength in the other muscles in the body, which brings stability.

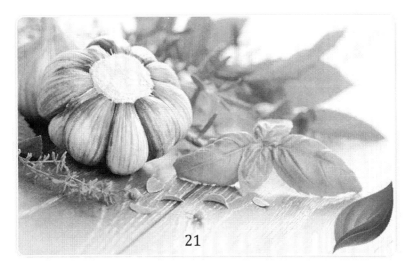

HEARTBURN

The best way to prevent heartburn is by maintaining a healthy weight and quitting smoking. Heartburn occurs when the esophageal sphincter loosens and causes stomach acid to back into the esophagus. Heartburn is characterized by a burning sensation in your chest and can be prevented by limiting certain foods and beverages such as caffeine, spicy and greasy foods as well as citrus fruit and tomatoes. However, when you are in the midst of experiencing heartburn, there are a few ways to find quick relief.

1.Baking Soda

Baking Soda, or sodium bicarbonate is naturally basic as it has a pH of 7.0 or higher. It neutralizes the stomach acid and provides instant relief.

Ingredients:
1 tsp. of baking soda
1 cup of filtered water

Directions:
Mix 1 tsp. of baking soda with 1 cup of filtered water thoroughly and drink the mixture when experiencing heartburn. You may repeat this remedy a couple of times daily but do not drink more than 3 teaspoons of baking soda in 24 hours or for longer than a period of one week as baking soda

has a high salt content and may produce swelling or nausea.

2. Aloe Juice

The Aloe Vera plant has incredible healing capacity, as you will learn in later chapters. Aloe Vera juice however, can also be incredibly beneficial in alleviating heartburn by reducing inflammation.

Directions:
Drink ½ cup of chilled Aloe Vera juice before meals. Because Aloe Vera juice can act as a laxative, make sure you choose a brand that has the laxative part removed.

Chapter 2

SKIN AND EXTERIOR BODY AILMENT REMEDIES

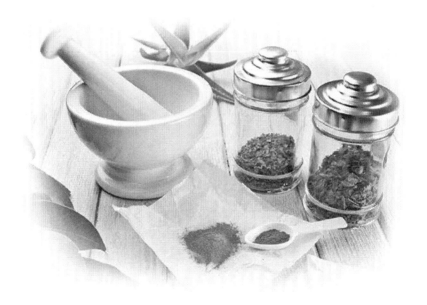

TOENAIL FUNGUS

Onychomycosis, or toenail fungus, is quite common. The toenail swells, inflames, yellows, crumbles, or thickens, and oftentimes the nail begins to crack. The fungus thrives under the skin's abnormal pH levels, a continued exposure to a humid environment, a weakened immune system, diabetes, and poor habits with regards to sock-cleaning and hygiene. Although it is not generally painful, toenail fungus is an unattractive situation, one that can eventually lead to loss of toenail.

1. Tea Tree Oil

Tea tree oil is utilized for toenail fungus due to its antifungal and antiseptic properties.

Directions:
Begin by mixing a few drops of the tea tree oil in a single teaspoon of either coconut oil or olive oil. Next, utilize a cotton ball to dose the affected toenail with the mixture. Allow the mixture to sit on the toenail for ten to fifteen minutes. Afterwards, scrub the toenail gently with a toothbrush. Operate in this manner three times a day until the required results are met.

2. Apple Cider Vinegar

Apple cider vinegar has an acidic base and therefore

eliminates the low pH problems associated with toenail fungus. Furthermore, it works to remove fungi and bacteria.

Directions:
Bring together ½ cup of apple cider vinegar and ½ cup of water. Place the toenail in the prepared solution for thirty minutes. Afterwards, dry the toenail gently but completely. Do this once a day for a number of weeks until the desired result is met.

3. Listerine Mouthwash

Listerine mouthwash is wonderful to use because it's generally found around the house. It kills the mouth's germs, and it can further eliminate fungus. Its several elements, like alcohol, have antiseptic qualities.

Directions:
Pour Listerine into a small bowl or tub. Place the affected toenail in the provided bowl and allow it to sit for thirty minutes. Afterwards, remove the infected toenail and scrub it gently with a toothbrush. Rinse the infected area and dry it completely. Utilize this technique twice a day to see results in about ten days.

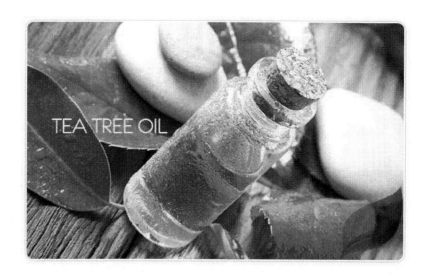

SUNBURN

An unfortunate misconception in popular culture is that one must be tan, a golden-brown that advertises happiness and health. Unfortunately, the road to this terrific suntan is wrought with flakey red skin and skin damage via that all-powerful entity: the sun. But overexposure to the sun can be met with natural home remedies; eliminate pain and stay comfortable with the following natural techniques.

1. Oatmeal Bath

Just as oatmeal assisted with skin pain from chicken pox in kindergarten, it can further offer reprieve from the pain of sunburns.

Directions:
Fill a bathtub with cool water. Make sure it's not cold water; cold water can shock the body. When the bath is full, scoop a full cup of oatmeal into the bath. Be sure not to utilize any oils, bath salts, or bubble bath when preparing the bath as these can irritate the skin further. Soak in the oatmeal bath for about fifteen to twenty minutes. Any longer than twenty minutes will dry the skin out. After exiting the bath, allow the skin to air-dry. Don't wipe the oatmeal from the skin with a towel.

2. Aloe Vera

Aloe Vera is found in countless over-the-counter sunburn remedies. However, Aloe Vera is actually a plant that can be easily purchased from a local grocery store's floral center. The juice from the inside of the stem removes redness and pain from a sunburn and allows blood vessels to constrict on the interior of the skin.

Directions:

Remove a broad leaf from the Aloe Vera plant and slit it open carefully. Slide the gel from the Aloe Vera leaf over the sunburn. Apply the gel five or six times each day for up to five days to eliminate pain entirely.

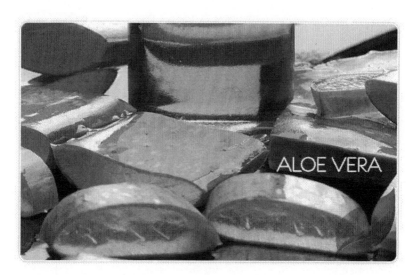

3. The Potato Method

Looking to potatoes for pain relief is actually a time-tested maneuver. They're used all over the world for exterior pain.

Directions:

Slice and dice two completely clean potatoes. Place the pieces in a blender or food processor and blend until they are a liquid. If they're a bit dry, add a little water. Take a bit of the potato mixture and pat on the affected area. Allow the potato to dry on the sunburn. Afterwards, take a short, cool shower. Use this method twice a day for four to five days to feel ultimate relief.

RASH

A skin rash is an outbreak of red, scaly bumps and can result from several conditions: outdoor allergens, food allergens, infections, etc. The rash is either widespread or localized, and it generally tingles, itches, blisters, or simply exists without pain. Allergic skin reactions are either systemic or dermal. Dermal skin rashes stem from direct contact with a specific allergen, while systemic skin rashes stem from food ingestion. Generally, systemic allergies are difficult to understand; however, the most common allergens are milk, eggs, soy, seafood, peanuts, and wheat. The most common dermal skin allergens are pollens, smoke, dust, lotions, soap products, and perfumes. Look to the following rash remedies for relief.

1. Raw Apple Cider Vinegar and Raw, Local Honey

Note: This technique is best utilized to eliminate allergies and thus eliminate rashes from the inside out.

Directions:

Bring together one tablespoon of raw, local honey, and one tablespoon of apple cider vinegar. Eat this small amount every day, three times a day to eliminate the body's reaction to certain exterior allergens. With this natural remedy, the body's allergic reaction in the form of a rash will fade away.

2. Poppy Seeds

Directions:
Crush one tablespoon of poppy seeds and mix the poppy seeds with a teaspoon of water. Add an additional teaspoon of lime juice. Mix. Apply the mixture to the rash twice a day until the rash begins to fade.

3. Basil Leaves

Directions:
Place three holy basil leaves, 2 garlic cloves, 1 tablespoon of olive oil, ½ teaspoon of salt, and ½ teaspoon of pepper in a food processor. Blend the ingredients well until they become a 'smearable' mixture. Place the mixture over the rash about twice a day until the rash begins to disappear.

ECZEMA

Eczema is a rash and flaking of the skin that develops due to environmental factors or diet and lifestyle factors. It is uncomfortable, quite itchy, and unattractive. The skin begins to look thickened, incredibly dry, and scale-like. Before applying the following home remedies, look to the soap and shampoo labels already in the shower. Read the ingredients. If the ingredients list something called: sodium laurel sulphate, throw the shampoo or soap away immediately. This is helping to boost eczema growth.

1. Magnesium Bath

Directions:
Bring together 2 cups magnesium flakes, ½ cup sea salt, ½ tsp. of vanilla extract and about fifteen drops of a favorite, calming essential oil. Try lavender or mint for the best stress eliminating remedy because stress is another central cause of eczema. Prepare a medium temperature bath and pour the mixture into it, allowing it to assimilate into the water. Soak in the bath for fifteen to twenty minutes. Remember: drying out the affected area is actually a good mechanism with regards to eczema. Therefore, a long bath is all right, as well.

2. Sweet Almond Carrier Oil

Sweet almond carrier oil is stocked with vitamins and plant compounds like oleic acid and ursolic acid. Both contain skin barrier repair effects and anti-inflammatory properties.

Directions:
Smear the sweet almond carrier oil over the affected eczema area and allow it to sit for sixty minutes. Afterwards, prepare a bath and soak for fifteen to twenty minutes, making sure not to utilize any soaps, shampoos, or bubble baths.

3. Coconut Oil

Coconut oil is essential for reduction of eczema. Because of its medium-chain fatty acids, it can assist with cell repair when applied topically, and it can bring about better gut health when digested. Because eczema has been linked with interior gut problems, it's best to begin cooking with coconut oil to provide an attack on all sides.

Directions:
Apply a thin layer of coconut oil over eczema to alleviate pain and itch. Do this approximately three times a day during flare-ups, and just once a day during non-flare up days. This way, eczema can be stopped at the source.

PSORIASIS

Psoriasis is a chronic skin disease consisting of scaly patches, plaque, redness, and papules. It generally itches, and can vary from small patches to total body coverage. Five main types of psoriasis include: inverse, plaque, guttate, erythrodermic, and pustular. Plaque is the most common version of psoriasis and occurs in white and red scales on the skin's exterior. Unfortunately, no complete cure is available for psoriasis. However, look to the following natural remedies to escape the discomfort and embarrassment of bad symptoms.

1. Turmeric

Turmeric is an anti-inflammatory substance utilized in India for thousands of years. Research shows that Curcumin, the active ingredient in the substance, can further alter gene expression; therefore, the substance has the ability to alter the skin's properties to reduce psoriasis flares.

Directions:
Turmeric comes in pill form, but it can also be added to foods like curry for maximum taste and digestive needs. Research shows that psoriasis and gut health are linked. Therefore, eating turmeric is one of the very essential ways one can reduce psoriasis symptoms. Note: the FDA states that 1.5 to 3.0 grams of turmeric is a safe amount.

2. Aloe Vera

As mentioned in the sunburn section, Aloe Vera has incredible benefits for the skin. The plant can be purchased in the local grocery store's plant section for the most natural benefits.

Directions:
Slice open a thick Aloe Vera leaf and apply the gel to the psoriasis affected area of the skin. Apply up to three times a day for maximum benefits; research states that scaling and redness associated with psoriasis can be dramatically reduced.

3. Sun Bathing

Sunlight is an incredibly, free natural remedy associated with psoriasis. 80% of people with psoriasis state their psoriasis improves with regular sunlight. Make sure to receive regular, brief amounts of sunlight every day. Sunburn tends to worsen psoriasis, and therefore it is recommended to always wear sunscreen on unaffected areas of the skin.

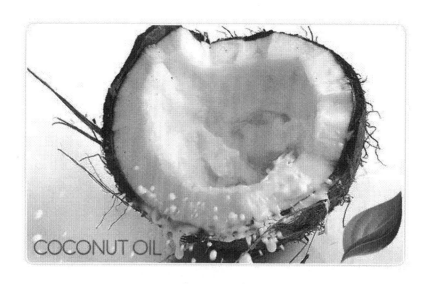

TIRED, PUFFY EYES

Personal appearance affects life in a number of different ways, and everyone wants to feel their best all the time. Puffy eyes from too much crying, too much physical strain or stress, hangovers, bad diet, lack of sleep, or hormonal changes can make one feel a little "off." Look to the following home remedies to eliminate tired eyes and recharge for the day ahead.

1. Tea Bags

Both green tea bags and black tea bags can soothe puffy, tired, and irritated eyes. Each contains anti-irritant properties and relieves interior inflammation.

Directions:

Begin by soaking two teabags, either black or green, in hot water for five minutes. Afterwards, remove the teabags from the water and allow them to cool to a subtle warmth. Next, lie down and place the tea bags over the eyes, covering them with a cloth. Lay just like that, relaxed, for about ten minutes. Repeat each morning as needed.

2. Chilled Cucumber

Cucumbers are stocked with enzymes and astringent properties, bringing a reduction of inflammation to the area around the eyes.

Directions:

Begin by slicing a cucumber into thick slices. Place the cucumber slices in the refrigerator for a full ten minutes. Afterwards, put one slice of cucumber over each eye and lay down for ten minutes. Repeat several times a day for a reduction of wrinkles and a brighter, daily outlook.

3. Egg Whites

The skin-tightening properties of egg whites lend added relief to the area around the eyes and further prevent wrinkles.

Directions:

Separate the egg whites from the yolks very carefully. Whip the egg whites with a whisk or a mixer. The consistency should be stiff. Afterwards, add a few drops of witch hazel to the egg whites. This allows for greater skin-tightening astringent. Apply the witch hazel and egg white mixture to the area under and around the eyes with a brush or a cloth. Allow the mixture to dry.

4. Potato

The starch of potatoes has intense anti-inflammatory properties that eliminate puffy eyes.

Directions:

Peel a well-cleaned potato and wash it. Afterwards, grate the potato and place the gratings in a clean cloth. Tie up the cloth and place it over the eyes for ten minutes. Repeat the potato process every morning or evening to cure eye puffiness.

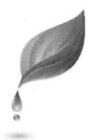

Chapter 3

GASTROINTESTINAL AILMENT REMEDIES

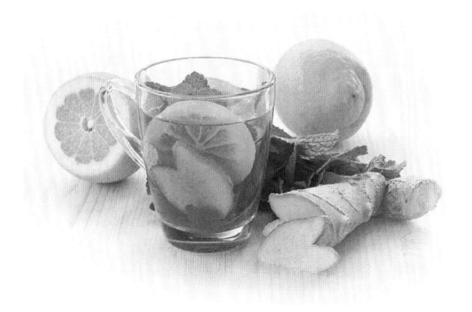

NAUSEA

Nausea is that feeling of sickness and unease accompanied, quite often, with vomiting. One can feel dizzy, uncomfortable, and often out-of-the-game for a few days. Nausea has a number of causes: from medications to morning sickness to motion sickness. Look to the natural remedies outlined below to eliminate sickness and get back into the world, rejuvenated. Remember that home remedies, especially in the case of nausea, are often better than over the counter medications. Over the counter medications often bring strong ingredients that further create interior unrest.

1. Milk and Toast

Bread and milk are often recommended to alleviate nausea symptoms. Milk coats the stomach, pushing back against acidity, while bread actually absorbs the excess stomach acid. Oftentimes, however, milk by itself can irritate the stomach. Therefore, milk toast is a go-to with nausea problems. Make sure, however, to avoid this if stomach flu, or gastroenteritis, is the reason behind the nausea. Dairy, unfortunately, irritates stomach flu.

Ingredients:
1 piece of toast
1 cup of milk
unsalted butter

Directions:

Heat a cup of milk in a saucepan until it's hot; make sure it doesn't turn to a boil. Pour the milk into a cereal bowl. Afterwards, toast a piece of bread and spread unsalted butter on the bread. Crumble the buttered toast into the bowl and eat the bread and milk with a spoon slowly.

2. Peppermint

Peppermint has a remarkable scent that can actually cut through nausea and ease an upset stomach.

Directions:

Place a bit of peppermint oil on a cotton swab and apply the swab directly on the gums. Reapply every few hours to eliminate all signs of nausea.

3. The BRAT Diet

Look to the BRAT diet to alleviate symptoms of nausea. So many different foods can actually churn nausea forward and irritate the stomach lining further. The BRAT diet, however, can keep everything under control.

Directions:

Eat the following foods: Bananas, Unsweetened Applesauce, Rice, and Toast. BRAT. Repeat until the stomach accepts vegetables again. Note: avoid vegetables at all cost until the nausea passes.

4. Ginger Tea

Ginger is a guaranteed natural remedy to halt nausea. It allows the digestive tract to secrete enzymes that actually neutralize stomach acid. Furthermore, it contains phenols, which allow the stomach muscles to relax. In addition, the phenols pulse the intestines, removing toxins more quickly. Ginger can be imbibed in several different ways: capsule form, raw root, or grated in soup. Look to the following tea recipe for immediate relief.

Directions:
Slice a two-inch, peeled ginger root into small sections. Cover it with wax paper and crush it for miniscule pieces. Bring 3 cups of water to a bowl in a sauce pan, and then place the ginger in the water, as well. Allow the ginger to boil for five minutes. Afterwards, remove the tea from the heat and drink slowly. Add honey for a bit of added sweetness.

CONSTIPATION

Constipation isn't a regular conversation topic, but boy can it ruin one's day. Don't rush to the store and buy any sort of laxatives, however. Laxatives can actually worsen the problems. And with several at-home remedies ready and available around the house, constipation should be out of the way in no time.

1. Olive Oil

Olive oil is pulsing with tasty, healthy fat, and it sparks the digestive system to get moving. If one utilizes olive oil regularly, one can actually prevent future bouts of constipation. Say goodbye to constipation and discomfort!

Directions:

Every morning, consume one tablespoon of olive oil and 1 teaspoon of lemon juice, mixed together. Eat this before eating anything else as it works best on an empty stomach. If the early morning is a forgetful time, wait to take the olive oil and lemon juice together a few hours after lunch, when the stomach is quite empty before dinner.

2. Blackstrap Molasses

Chronic and occasional constipation alike can look to the benefits of blackstrap molasses for relief. Regular molasses is simple cane sugar boiled until the sugar is concentrated and crystallized. Blackstrap molasses results after the third boiling. The crystallization results in several vitamins and minerals. Magnesium, one of these minerals, revs the digestive system. Best of all, blackstrap molasses is delicious and natural.

Directions:
Every morning before consuming any breakfast items, consume one teaspoon of blackstrap molasses. If the flavor of molasses doesn't suit, place the teaspoon of molasses in warm water and drink it that way. If one teaspoon lacks any sort of effectiveness in the body, work up to one or two tablespoons.

3. Natural Fiber

Natural diets relieve constipation—the natural way. Look to fruits, grains, and vegetables before even taking a peek at any of that artificial, processed stuff. The body understands how to digest natural elements from these foods, and thus revs the digestive system forward, promoting the colon's processes.

Directions:
Eat good fiber-stocked foods like: Plums, apples, pears, broccoli, apricots, nuts, beans, whole grain bread, and berries.

Note: Avoid over-consumption of beans. Beans are full of fiber; however, they can occasionally contribute to constipation without enough inclusion of water in the diet.

4. Flaxseed Oil

Flaxseed oil is an oft-sought remedy for constipation. It works to coat the walls of the intestines to increase bowel movements.

Directions:
Bring together eight ounces of orange juice and one tablespoon of flaxseed oil. Mix the two together well and drink slowly.

Note: Oranges are further stocked with fiber, making this drink an excellent constipation relief. Remember that the drink will take a few hours to work; therefore, don't dare drink another mixture for at least eight hours after the first.

5. Aloe Vera

The Aloe Vera skin benefits are undeniable and written about time and time again in this book. However, Aloe Vera further soothes constipation and allows the body to revert back to natural processes. Find the Aloe Vera plant in the grocery store plant department; alternately, look to the Aloe Vera juice found in a natural health food store.

Process:
Remove an Aloe Vera plant leaf from the plant and slice it open to reveal the gel-like substance on the interior. Remove two tablespoons of the gel substance from the plant and place it in one glass of any kind of fruit juice. Stir well and drink in the morning, before eating any sort of breakfast meal.

6. Baking Soda

Baking soda is the secret little trinket to alleviate so many nasty body problems. And there it is: found inside kitchen cabinets all over the world! It is a bicarbonate, and is therefore able to encourage the removal of air from the body in any way possible. Therefore, the pressure building in the stomach and intestines will be relieved. Furthermore, baking soda neutralizes the stomach acid and allows for proper digestion.

Directions:
Bring together a teaspoon of baking soda and ¼ cup of warm water. Drink the mixture quickly. The baking soda will not take long to initiate in the stomach.

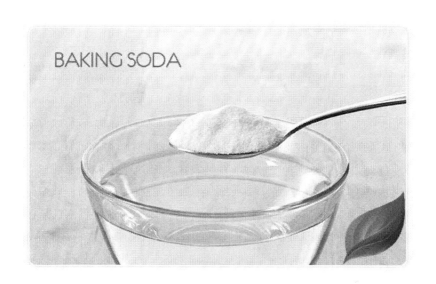

DIARRHEA

When diarrhea strikes, it can wreck real havoc on your daily life. Not only is this condition uncomfortable and painful, it can be embarrassing as well. The following are proven ways to provide relief from diarrhea and restore health to your intestinal lining.

1. Make Sure to Stay Hydrated

Loss of water and electrolytes is a common side effect of diarrhea and can lead to mild, moderate, or severe dehydration. Common signs of dehydration include dry eyes, skin and mucous membranes, severe thirst, sunken eyes as well as confusion and irritability. Drink 8-12 cups of chilled water daily to replenish lost fluids. Sip instead of guzzling down for increased absorption; this is easier on your stomach.

2. Eat Live Culture Yogurt

Consuming a couple of servings of plain, pro-biotic yogurt provides protection to your intestinal lining, the "good bacteria' produce lactic acid which kills off harmful bacteria in your intestines. Therefore, probiotic yogurt replenishes the "healthy" bacteria and this is especially important if you are taking antibiotics.

3. Drink Mint Tea

Drink 4-6 cups of freshly brewed mint tea daily to alleviate diarrhea. For optimal results, buy 4-5 stalks of fresh mint at your local supermarket. Wash thoroughly and roll the stalks of mint between the palms of your hands to release the oils. Place the mint in a teapot and pour 4 cups of boiling water over the mint stalks. Wait 5 minutes for the tea to steep. Sip on the mint tea slowly.

4. Use a Heating Pad

If you are experiencing abdominal cramps, try placing a heating pad over your abdomen for pain relief.

5. Avoid Certain Foods

Avoid the following foods as they may worsen the symptoms of diarrhea:
Milk and dairy products
Alcohol
Greasy and spicy foods
Caffeine

BLOATING AND GAS

Bloating and gas are commonly experienced together and most often are the result of eating certain foods but may have many different causes. As uncomfortable and embarrassing as they may be, there are ways in which you can alleviate most of the unpleasant discomfort.

1. Peppermint tea

As already mentioned, peppermint tea is great for soothing your tummy. It contains methanol, which is an essential oil and has an antispasmodic response on the muscle in your digestive tract.

Ingredients:
1 cup of boiling water
1 bag of peppermint tea

Directions:
Boil water and pour into a mug over the peppermint tea. Let steep for 5 minutes and enjoy.

2. Ginger

Again, ginger is great for nausea and upset stomach in general but it also works great with bloating and gas. It contains chemicals that assist in decreasing the inflammation in the digestive tract. Aside from that it also helps to prevent and expel gas because it acts as a carminative.

Ingredients:
1 inch of grated ginger root
1 cup water
Lemon and honey

Directions:
Wash and scrub the ginger root before grating it.
Heat water and pour over freshly grated ginger root
(it does not need to be boiled). Add lemon and
honey to taste, cover and steep for 10 minutes.
Drink 1 cup before or after a meal to prevent gas and
aid in digestion.

3. Caraway Seeds

Caraway seeds have been used to eliminate trapped
gas out of the digestive tract for centuries. They are
abundant in vitamins and minerals and have
powerful carminative properties that release
trapped gas and prevent the formation of gas as
well.

Ingredients:
1 tsp. of caraway seeds

Directions:
Try snacking on a handful of caraway seeds or
caraway seed crackers when you are feeling bloated
or unable to pass gas. If this is a continuous problem
for you, try eating a small amount of caraway seeds

each morning before breakfast to prevent the formation of gas during the day.

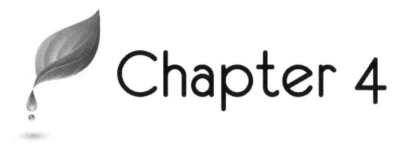

Chapter 4

MENTAL AND NEUROLOGICAL
AILMENT REMEDIES

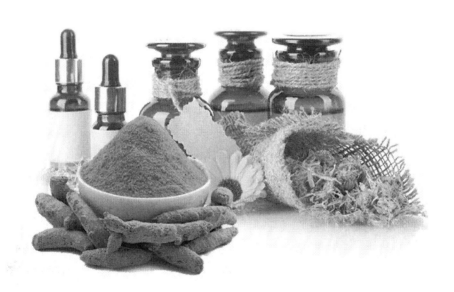

VERTIGO

Severe dizziness, life-altering symptoms: this is the reality of those experiencing vertigo. The causes of vertigo are quite complex; generally, dizziness and confusion occurs when one stands up too quickly or changes the position of one's head. However, recent research understands that at-home treatment is just as successful as doctor treatments. During the week after beginning a well-structured, quite simple physical therapy schedule in their home, 95% of vertigo patients experienced no dizziness.

Note: the following at-home techniques are for patients suffering from both benign paroxysmal positional vertigo and top-shelf vertigo. Top-shelf vertigo is generally found in patients over the age of seventy-five; it occurs when the patient looks up or down, altering the head position.

1. Physical Therapy

Directions:
Begin by sitting on the bed and placing a pillow directly behind the back. While still sitting up, turn the head 45 degrees to the right if the vertigo exists in the right ear. Alternately, turn the head 45 degrees to the left if the vertigo exists in the left ear. With the head still positioned this way, lie back on the pillow rapidly. The shoulders should fall on the pillow, the neck should be extended, and the head should be on the bed. The affected ear is on the bed.

Rest there for thirty seconds. Next, turn the head a full 90 degrees in the alternate direction and wait for an additional thirty seconds. After these thirty seconds, align the body this same direction and wait another thirty seconds. Sit up with the head facing in the opposite direction from which it began.

This maneuver must be done a full three times a day until the vertigo disappears for a full twenty-four hours.

2. Ginger

Ginger tea strikes again in this remarkable home remedy. It's a traditional cure for motion sickness, dating back to the ages of long boat trips across the ocean.

Directions:

Bring two cups of water to a boil in a saucepan. Grate one inch of ginger over the water and allow the water to simmer for an additional five minutes. Afterwards, strain the tea and drink slowly.

3. Wheat Grain and Almond Paste

Ingredients:

2 tbsp. wheat grain
1 tsp. poppy seeds
8 watermelon seeds
8 almonds
1 tsp. ghee
2 cloves

Directions:

Soak 1 teaspoon of poppy seeds, 2 tablespoons of wheat grain, 8 watermelon seeds, and 8 almonds together in 1/2 cup of water. After they've soaked for two hours, place the mixture in a food processor and make a paste. To the side in a saucepan, heat 1 tsp. ghee and 2 cloves. After it's heated on medium-high heat for five minutes, add the ghee and cloves to the paste and mix once more. Drink this paste every single day for a week or until vertigo symptoms pass.

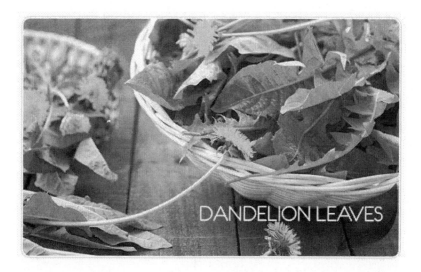

DANDELION LEAVES

ANXIETY

The world is often a difficult place to maneuver. Anxiety, in the form of rapid, shallow breathing, imagined doom, and inability to relax, haunts people of all ages, in all stages. Rid panic without looking to drugs. Look to the following nondrug remedies to safely eliminate anxiety and get back to life.

1. Chamomile Tea

Incredibly, chamomile compounds bind to the same brain receptors that prescription drug Valium binds to, thus calming the "racing thoughts" aspect of anxiety. A recent study out of Pennsylvania Medical Center in Philadelphia found that patients with anxiety disorders who stocked themselves with chamomile supplements every day for eight weeks had an incredible decrease in symptoms from anxiety.

Directions:
Steep a cup of boiling water with two tablespoons of dried chamomile leaves for ten minutes, covered. Remove the cover and strain the tea. Enjoy slowly, calmly.

2. L-theanine in Green Tea

Green tea contains an amino acid called L-theanine that produces soothing and calming effects. According to new research, this amino acid helps to slow the heart rate and the blood pressure, resulting in calm feelings.

Directions:
Drink four to six mugs of green tea every single day to curb anxiety.

3. Eat a Balanced Diet

Generally speaking, hungry people are anxious people. Their blood sugar is dropping, and they required a snack of some sort. Next time anxiety takes its toll, look to a few walnuts, almonds, a piece of dark chocolate, or a cup of tea. Remember that an everyday diet warrants whole foods, plant-based foods, and meats and seafood. Phytonutrients stocked in leafy greens help eliminate anxiety.

MILD DEPRESSION

Mild depression affects approximately ten percent of adults; it renders itself with feelings of anger, sadness, and frustration. Mild-depression can continue for weeks, affecting all parts of work and personal life. Most often, mild depression is triggered by stressful experiences or chronic pain. Note: In the event of persistent and chronic depression and suicidal thoughts please seek medical advice and treatment.

1. Omega-3 Fatty Acids

Research states that omega-3 fatty acids from cold water fish like salmon and tuna are absolutely necessary for the regulation of the neural passageways. If one of these passageways is affected it can alter one's mood. The brain is a full sixty percent fat, and much of this fat is omega-3 fatty acids. The omega-3 fatty acids are crucial in promoting cell-to-cell communication. Because scientists believe that depression finds its root in poor brain chemical signals, omega-3 fatty acid boosts can eliminate these problems. Consume a diet rich in omega-3 fatty acids. Rich sources include flax seeds, walnuts, sardines, salmon, Brussels sprouts, cauliflower and winter squash.

2. Stock Up on Folic Acid

Folic acid is a B vitamin generally lacking in

depressed people. Find folic acid in beans, fruit, green leafy vegetables, and grains. A recent Harvard study noted that depressed people with low amounts of folic acid didn't respond well to anti-depressants. Therefore, boosting folic acid could be a better remedy than chemically altering drugs.

3. St. John's Wort

St. John's Wort is an ancient herb long used in folk medicine for worry, nerves, sadness, and insomnia. Recent trials suggest that St. John's Wort matches anti-depressant results without the added side effects. Find St. John's Wort in a local health food store in tablet, capsule, or tea formation. After four to six weeks, a dramatic increase of mood should occur.

4. Exercise

Exercise is the most underutilized natural remedy for depression we know of today. When you exercise, you produce endorphins, "the feel good" chemicals in the brain and decrease the stress hormone, cortisol, circulating in your body. There are numerous research studies that show that exercising can be as effective in treating various forms of depression as some of the commonly used antidepressants on the market today. In addition, exercise doesn't produce any negative side effects and helps with elevating your mood, decreasing anxiety, reducing insomnia and much more.

Engage in 30 min of moderate physical activity 3 times per week. This can include biking, running, swimming, jogging, or any other activity that gets your heart going.

INSOMNIA

Adults need about seven to nine hours of sleep every single night in order for all body processes to operate correctly. And yet: insomnia also affects something like one-third of all adults. Sleepless nights force one into mediocre days, days without a reach toward one's potential. With insomnia, one is four times more likely to be depressed, far more likely to have an accident on the road, and more likely to have a serious illness. Despite the fact that insomnia is not very well understood, sleep experts understand a few natural remedies to work back to nights full of sleep. Look to the following remedies to rejuvenate once more.

1. Limit Both Alcohol and Caffeine

When the alcohol consumption begins, one actually begins to feel drowsy. However, once that drowsiness turns to sleep, one is naturally more likely to wake up in a few hours with a full bladder, a headache, or a stomachache. Caffeine, on the other hand, stimulates one's brain, disallowing sleep. After noon, consume nothing caffeinated.

2. Eat a Bit of Sugar

One should generally stop eating a few hours before bedtime to allow the digestive system to calm down and begin repairing itself during the evening hours. However, a bit of sugar thirty minutes prior to sleep can actually allow one to sleep soundly throughout the night. Look to something small and healthy, like a bit of honey in some herbal tea or warm milk.

3. Aromatherapy

English lavender has been utilized as a folk sleep remedy for hundreds of years. It soothes and relaxes in the hours before bedtime. Lavender essential oil lengthens sleep time, helps one to feel more refreshed in the morning hours, and increases the length of deep sleep.

Directions:
Place a lavender sachet under a pillow before you go to sleep. Alternately, drip two drops of lavender essential oil on a cloth and place it beneath the pillow. A warm bath with a few drops of lavender essential oil calms, as well, and adds some wonderful aromatherapy for the senses.

4. Chamomile Tea

Chamomile is a particular stress-relieving herb. When brewed in tea, it reduces muscle tension, reduces anxiety, and soothes digestion, thereby allowing increased ability for sound sleep. Passionflower, hops, and ashwagandha are other excellent herbs that hold the same effects as chamomile.

5. Gentle Music

Listening to soft, soothing music in the hour prior to sleep can calm and allow one to improve sleep quality. Furthermore, music can decrease middle of the night wakening and increase one's satisfaction.

Chapter 5

INFECTION AILMENT REMEDIES

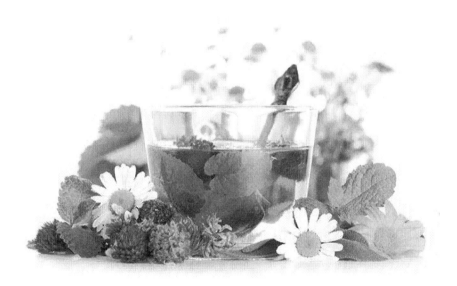

FIRST AID OINTMENT

Scratches and scrapes are the simple result of living life out loud. Allow the body to repair with a boost from the following natural remedies; don't look to the ingredient-laden creams and ointments at the local pharmacy.

1. Yarrow and Calendula First Aid Ointment

Yarrow allows the body to stop bleeding and works to eliminate insects surrounding the damaged area. Calendula, on the other hand, is a remarkable, essential healing herb with anti-inflammatory properties.

Ingredients:
¼ cup Calendula petals
¼ cup comfrey
2 tbsp. arnica
¼ cup yarrow flower
1 ½ cup coconut oil
5 drops lavender essential oil
5 drops melaleuca essential oil
2 tbsp. beeswax

Directions:
Begin by preheating the oven to 200 degrees Fahrenheit. Pour coconut oil into a medium-sized saucepan and heat over medium heat until it's completely melted. Afterwards, add the herbs: the Calendula petals, the comfrey, the arnica, and the

yarrow flowers. Stir well for two minutes.

Next, remove the saucepan and pour the contents into a small baking dish. Place the baking dish in the preheated oven and then completely turn off the oven. Walk away for a few hours—about three or four.

Remove the herbs and oil from the oven and strain the oil into a measuring cup. After straining, add a little more coconut oil so that you have a full 1 and ½ cups. When the measuring cup is filled with 1 ½ cups coconut oil, pour the coconut oil with infused herbs back into the saucepan and heat over medium. Add the beeswax and allow it to melt.

After the beeswax has melted, remove the mixture from the heat and allow it to cool. Pour the cooled mixture into cleaned jars and store the jars in a cool location. Rub the ointment on any cuts or scrapes as needed.

2. Plantain Salve Remedy

Plantain is occasionally referred to as the "band aid" plant. It's stocked with something called iridoid, which is an incredible anti-inflammatory that provides a soothing remedy. Furthermore, it features aucubigenin and aglycone, both of which display antimicrobial effects.

Ingredients:
1 cup plantain leaves
1 ½ cups coconut oil
1 ½ tbsp. beeswax
1 tsp. rosemary essential oil

Directions:
Make sure prior to utilizing the following recipe that the plantain leaves are incredibly dry. Leaves with dampness to them won't last quite as long due to their affinity for bacteria.

Chop the plantain leaves or place them in a food processor. Grind them, and pour them into a mason jar. Cover the leaves with liquid coconut oil. The oil should cover the plantain leaves completely.

Next, align a towel at the bottom of the crockpot and place the covered jar on the towel in the crockpot. Add water to the crock up to align it at the halfway mark of the jar. Set the crockpot to the lowest setting and allow it to heat for twenty-four hours.

Afterwards, remove the oil jar from the crockpot and strain the oil. Allow the oil to sit in a cool, dark place for four hours. Any additional water from the plantain leaves will collect at the bottom of the oil, perfect for removal.

Next, place the beeswax in a medium-sized bowl. Place that bowl in a pre-boiling, large pan of water.

Allow the beeswax to melt. After it's melted, add the plantain oil—without the collected water at the bottom. Stir the plantain oil and the beeswax together. Remove the mixture from the heat and allow it to cool to the side. When it's cooled, drip the rosemary essential oils into the mixture and stir well. Store the salve in a dry container and place it in a cool, dark place. Prepare for any and all bug bites, bee stings, cuts, and scrapes.

COMMON COLD

The common cold doesn't feel so common. Out for the count, people are stuck with a cough, a stuffy nose, a headache, constant muscle aches, and a sore throat. Millions of people spend countless amounts of money on cold remedies. However, there's not a single cure for the common cold on the market. That's because a cold is an upper-respiratory infection caused by a broad number of viruses. Look to the following at-home remedies to recover and get back into the world.

1. Saline Drops

Inflammation in the nose is caused by cytokines or lymphokines, which are molecules made by the body to stomp infection. However, research understands that eliminating these molecules can help with reducing nose swelling and discomfort.

Directions:
Make saline drops by simply adding ¼ teaspoon of salt to eight ounces of distilled water. Place the mixture in a nasal spray and spray in the nostrils three times, six times a day.

2. Eat Hot Peppers

Hot peppers force the eyes to water and the nose to run. They contain capsaicin which is similar to guaifenesin, a component found in cough syrups. Therefore, they are great assistants in clearing the stuffy nose of meddlesome mucus. Heat up some hot peppers and spice up the next meal for added relief.

3. Load Up on Vitamin C

Munching on Vitamin C-stocked foods won't necessarily prevent the common cold. However, research shows that loading up on vitamin C during cold-times can help strengthen the immune system and cut down on the sickness time. Boosting vitamin intake to reduce cold symptoms, however, requires about 2,000 mg of Vitamin C, an incredible leap from the ordinary recommended dosage of 60 mg. Research shows that taking a lot of vitamin C for a short time is not harmful; however, prolonged vitamin C intake can result in severe diarrhea.

Stock up on citrus foods like lemons, oranges, limes, and grapefruits. Drink vitamin-C stocked juice.

4. Sleep with Two Pillows

Placing an extra pillow beneath the head during sleep can assist with clearing nasal passageways as it changes the angle of the nostrils, pushing blood flow away. If the angle of a second pillow is difficult to maintain, place a pillow beneath the mattress for a more aligned, gradual slope.

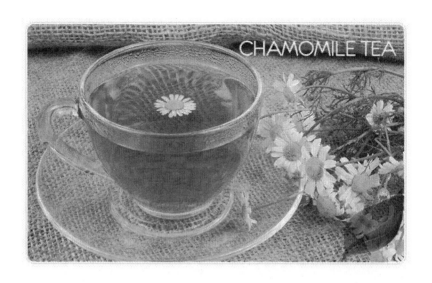

1. Natural Honey and Apple Cider Vinegar Cough Syrup Recipe

Honey is a natural cough suppressant, and apple cider vinegar holds intense antiseptic properties.

Directions:
Make at-home cough syrup by mixing together ¼ cup apple cider and ¼ cup honey. Stir well, and store the mixture in a jar. Shake well prior to using, and take just one tablespoon every four hours until coughing subsides.

2. Thyme Leaves Tea

In Germany, thyme is regarded as an official treatment for upper respiratory infections, coughs, and whopping cough. Each leaf is stocked with anti-cough compounds. Flavanoids relax both the ileal muscles and the tracheal muscles. Furthermore, the leaves reduce inflammation.

Directions:
Crush two teaspoons of thyme leaves and place them in a cup of boiling water. Cover the water for ten minutes and strain prior to enjoying. Enjoy three times a day until coughing subsides.

3. Flaxseed, Lemon, and Honey Cough Remedy

The gooey creation formed with flaxseed, lemon, and honey soothes both the bronchial tract and the throat. The lemon and honey serve as antibiotics and bring a sweet, sunny taste to the mixture.

Directions:
Place three tablespoons of flaxseed in a cup of water. Boil the water until the mixture becomes frothy and thick. Next, strain the water and add three tablespoons of lemon juice and three tablespoons of honey. Take it a tablespoon at a time, three times a day until coughing subsides.

4. Black Pepper Tea

Black pepper tea is a mainstay in both Chinese medicine and New England folk medicine. Black pepper is said to stimulate mucus flow and circulation, while honey is a general cough reliever. Note: this cough reliever is most optimal for wet coughs.

Directions:
Pour one teaspoon of fresh, ground black pepper into a cup. Add two tablespoons of honey and stir. Next, pour boiling water into the cup and allow the mixture to steep for a full fifteen minutes, covered. Strain the pepper a bit, and drink as needed throughout the day to reduce inflammation and coughing.

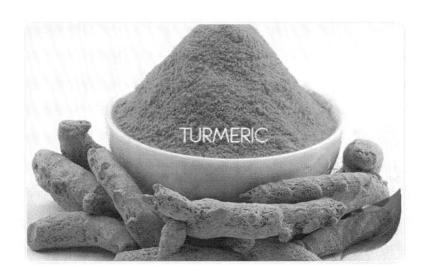

SORE THROAT

A sore throat oftentimes accompanies a terrible flu or a cold and can make your life miserable. As already mentioned, although there is no cure for a cold or for sore throat for that matter, there are natural ways in which you can alleviate the soreness and pain:

1. Salt Water

As your grandmother probably told you, salt water can work wonders on your throat. During an infection, your cells get swollen and inflamed and more mucous is produced. Salt water helps to draw water out of the cells therefore helping to reduce the swelling and inflammation. It also helps to clear mucous membranes and will help with a runny nose.

Ingredients:
1 cup warm water
½ tsp. salt

Directions:
Boil water and wait until it's warm. Pour into a mug, add salt and mix well. Gargle 3 times daily for best results.

2. Lemon, Honey and Water

Lemon lends the much needed vitamin C and has cleansing and detoxifying properties while honey helps to soothe your throat.

Ingredients:

1 tbsp. honey

1 cup hot water

1 tbsp. lemon juice

1 slice of lemon

Directions:

Boil water and pour into a large cup; mix in the honey and lemon juice. Stir well. Add the lemon slice, sip and enjoy.

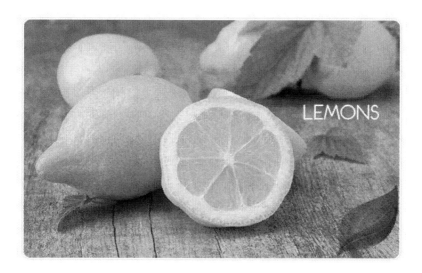

3. Apple Cider Vinegar and Honey

Apple Cider Vinegar is very acidic and therefore helps to kill the bacteria while honey helps to soothe your throat.

Ingredients:
1 cup of water
1 tbsp. of honey
1 tbsp. apple cider vinegar

Directions:
Boil water, pour into a cup and wait until it's warm. Stir in honey and apple cider vinegar. Mix well and enjoy once daily until soreness subsides.

Conclusion

Natural remedies allow you to look beyond the stocked walls of the local pharmacy; they allow you to eliminate chemicals and crazy ingredients from your everyday medicines. Look to the natural elements of the earth to work through the common cold, bug bites, and sunburns; alleviate common pains and work to rejuvenate your life with herbs, fruits and vegetables. This book holds a higher standard for life-affirming foods. You can with the use of natural remedies eliminate pain, save your money from the medicinal industry, and retreat to a safer, cleaner lifestyle once and for all.

Printed in Poland
by Amazon Fulfillment
Poland Sp. z o.o., Wrocław